JEREMY HAINES

Eat Clean Get Healthy Be Happy

A Guide to Health, Longevity and Happiness

This book was professionally typeset on Reedsy.
Find out more at reedsy.com

The Greatest Wealth is Health

-Virgil

Contents

1

Introduction

In a world inundated with quick fixes and fad diets promising instant results, the pursuit of optimal health and happiness can often feel like an elusive quest. However, nestled within the core principles of clean eating, lifestyle modifications, and sustainable weight loss lies a transformative journey toward holistic well-being.

"Eat Clean, Lose Weight, Be Happy" is not just another diet book; it's a comprehensive guide that delves into the intricate relationship between physical nourishment and mental vitality. Within these pages, we embark on a journey that transcends mere calorie counting and restrictive meal plans. Instead, we explore the profound impact of nutrition, mindful consumption, and positive lifestyle changes on both the body and the mind.

This book is a testament to the power of reclaiming control over our health and happiness through informed choices and intentional living. By embracing the principles of clean eating, we not only shed excess weight but also nourish our bodies with the vital nutrients they crave. Through mindfulness practices and stress management techniques, we cultivate resilience and emotional well-being in the face of life's challenges.

Drawing upon the latest research in nutrition, psychology, and holistic wellness, "Eat Clean, Lose Weight, Be Happy" offers practical strategies, delicious recipes, and actionable insights to empower you on your journey toward a healthier, happier life. Whether you're seeking to trim down, boost energy levels, or simply revitalise your outlook on life, this book serves as your trusted companion and roadmap to sustainable transformation.

As we embark on this transformative journey together, remember that true wellness extends beyond the numbers on a scale. It encompasses nourishing the body, nurturing the soul, and embracing the joy of living fully. So, let us embark on this journey together, one mindful bite at a time, as we discover the profound rewards of eating clean, losing weight, and embracing the boundless potential for happiness that resides within each of us.

2

Lifestyle Change For Longevity

In the pursuit of wellness, lifestyle change stands as the cornerstone for achieving sustainable health and vitality. Embracing a lifestyle oriented towards holistic well-being transcends diet and exercise; it encompasses a shift in mindset, habits, and environment. This section dives into the fundamental principles and practical strategies for initiating and sustaining lifestyle changes conducive to optimal health.

Understanding the Dynamics of Lifestyle Change

At its core, lifestyle change entails a deliberate departure from habits and patterns that compromise health, towards behaviours that promote vitality and longevity. Recognizing the interconnectedness of physical, mental, and emotional health is pivotal in fostering comprehensive lifestyle transformations. Embracing a growth mindset, characterised by openness to new experiences and resilience in the face of setbacks, forms the bedrock of sustainable change.

The Power of Habit Formation

Central to lifestyle modification is the cultivation of health-promoting habits. Harnessing the principles of behavioural psychology, individuals can systematically replace detrimental habits with positive ones. Leveraging cues, routines, and rewards, habit formation becomes a potent tool for instilling lasting behavioural changes. Whether it's adopting a consistent exercise regimen, prioritising nutritious meals, or cultivating mindfulness practices, the cumulative impact of small, incremental changes cannot be overstated.

Nutrition as Nourishment

A cornerstone of healthy living lies in mindful nutrition. Embracing a diet rich in whole, unprocessed foods serves as a potent catalyst for vitality and disease prevention. Prioritising plant-based fare abundant in colourful fruits, vegetables, legumes, and whole grains not only fuels the body with essential nutrients but also confers myriad health benefits. Cultivating mindful eating practices, such as savouring each bite and tuning into hunger cues, fosters a deeper connection with food and enhances digestive wellness.

Embracing Physical Activity

Regular exercise is indispensable in fostering physical resilience and emotional well-being. Engaging in a diverse array of activities, spanning cardiovascular, strength training, flexibility, and balance exercises, ensures comprehensive fitness and reduces the risk of chronic disease. Integrating movement into daily routines, whether through brisk walks, yoga sessions, or recreational sports, cultivates an active lifestyle tailored to individual preferences and capabilities.

Nurturing Emotional and Mental Wellness

True health encompasses emotional and mental equilibrium. Prioritising stress management techniques, such as meditation, deep breathing exercises, and expressive arts, fosters resilience in the face of life's challenges. Cultivating supportive social networks and fostering meaningful connections nourishes the soul and bolsters emotional well-being. Embracing self-compassion and cultivating a positive outlook imbues life with purpose and vitality.

Creating a Supportive Environment

Sustaining lifestyle changes necessitates a nurturing environment conducive to growth and flourishing. Surrounding oneself with supportive peers, mentors, and resources cultivates accountability and reinforces positive habits. Designing living and workspaces that prioritise health, such as incorporating greenery, natural light, and ergonomic design elements, fosters an environment conducive to well-being.

Conclusion: A Journey of Transformation

Embarking on a journey of lifestyle change is a profound act of self-care and empowerment. By embracing holistic principles and cultivating health-promoting habits, individuals forge a path towards vitality, resilience, and fulfilment. Through steadfast commitment, self-awareness, and a willingness to adapt, the pursuit of optimal health becomes not merely a destination, but a transformative journey imbued with purpose and possibility.

3

Whole Foods, Clean Eating and Balance

In our quest for healthier living, the terms "whole foods" and "clean eating" have gained prominence. But what do they really mean, and how can we integrate them into our lives without sacrificing our favourite indulgences? This chapter explores the essence of whole foods and clean eating, emphasising the importance of moderation in our dietary choices.

Understanding Whole Foods

Whole foods are as nature intended—minimally processed and close to their natural state. They retain their original nutrients, fibre, and health-promoting compounds. Think of vibrant fruits and vegetables, hearty whole grains, lean proteins, and wholesome nuts and seeds. Choosing whole foods means opting for ingredients that nourish our bodies without added sugars, artificial flavours, or preservatives.

The Principles of Clean Eating

Clean eating goes hand in hand with whole foods. It involves selecting foods that are nutrient-dense and free from unnecessary additives. Clean eating encourages consuming foods that support overall health and well-being. This includes prioritising organic produce, opting for lean proteins, and choosing whole grains over refined ones. The emphasis is on quality, freshness, and simplicity.

Moderation: The Key to Balance

While whole foods and clean eating form the foundation of a healthy diet, embracing moderation allows us to enjoy our favourite foods without guilt or restriction. Moderation is about finding balance—nourishing our bodies with nutrient-rich foods while savouring the occasional indulgence.

Moderation means enjoying that slice of decadent chocolate cake at a celebration or savouring a scoop of creamy gelato on a warm summer day. It's about sipping a glass of wine with friends or relishing a piece of cheese with crusty bread. Moderation doesn't mean deprivation; rather, it fosters a healthy relationship with food, where all foods have their place in a balanced diet.

Practical Tips for Whole Foods and Clean Eating with Moderation:

Fill Your Plate with Color

Aim to incorporate a variety of colourful fruits and vegetables into your meals. These nutrient-packed foods not only add flavour and texture but also provide essential vitamins and minerals.

Choose Whole Grains

Opt for whole grains like brown rice, quinoa, and oats over refined grains like white rice and white bread. Whole grains offer more fibre and nutrients, keeping you feeling fuller for longer.

Prioritise Lean Proteins

Include lean sources of protein such as poultry, fish, tofu, and legumes in your diet. These proteins provide essential amino acids for muscle repair and growth.

Read Labels Mindfully

When purchasing packaged foods, read labels carefully. Look for simple ingredients lists with recognizable items. Avoid products with added sugars, trans fats, and artificial additives.

Practise Mindful Eating

Slow down and savour each bite. Pay attention to hunger and fullness cues, eating until satisfied rather than stuffed. Mindful eating allows you to appreciate the flavours and textures of your food while fostering a healthier relationship with eating.

Embracing Whole Foods, Clean Eating, and Moderation

Whole foods and clean eating offer a roadmap to better health and vitality, while moderation ensures enjoyment and balance along the journey. By prioritising nutrient-rich foods and savouring indulgences in moderation, we can nourish our bodies and souls while embracing a sustainable approach to healthy living.

Remember, it's not about perfection but progress. Embrace the journey, savour the flavours, and celebrate the joy of nourishing your body and spirit with whole foods, clean eating, and the beautiful balance of moderation.

4

Longevity And Blue Zones

Blue zones are regions around the world where people tend to live significantly longer, healthier lives compared to the global average. These regions have attracted attention from researchers studying longevity and healthy ageing. The term "blue zones" was coined by Dan Buettner, a National Geographic Fellow, who identified five areas known for the longevity of their populations:

1. Ikaria, Greece

The mountainous Greek island of Ikaria has a high concentration of centenarians and low rates of chronic diseases like heart disease and cancer.

2. Okinawa, Japan

Okinawa is known for its high number of centenarians and a diet rich in vegetables, tofu, and fish, along with strong social support networks.

3. Sardinia, Italy

The mountainous region of Sardinia has a significant number of male centenarians, likely due to a combination of genetics, diet (rich in vegetables, legumes, and goat's milk), and lifestyle factors.

4. Nicoya Peninsula, Costa Rica

Residents of the Nicoya Peninsula have low rates of middle-age mortality and a strong sense of purpose, along with a diet high in beans, corn, and tropical fruits.

5. Loma Linda, California, USA**

Loma Linda is home to a community of Seventh-day Adventists who have longer life expectancy due to their plant-based diets, regular exercise, strong social networks, and religious beliefs.

The significance of blue zones lies in the insights they offer into the factors that contribute to longevity and overall well-being. Common characteristics observed in these regions include:

Diet

Blue zone residents typically follow plant-based diets rich in fruits, vegetables, whole grains, and legumes.

Physical activity

Daily physical activity, often integrated into daily routines, helps maintain health and vitality.

Social connections

Strong social support networks and a sense of belonging contribute to mental well-being and longevity.

Purpose

Having a sense of purpose and meaning in life has been linked to better health outcomes and longevity.

Stress management

Blue zone inhabitants often practise stress-relieving activities such as meditation, prayer, or taking regular breaks.

Studying blue zones has led to the development of health promotion initiatives and lifestyle interventions aimed at promoting longevity and well-being in other communities around the world.

5

Nourish Your Body The Right Way

Macronutrients and micronutrients play vital roles in maintaining overall health and supporting weight loss goals.

Macronutrients

Carbohydrates, Proteins, and Fats
These are the three macronutrients that provide energy (calories) and serve as building blocks for various bodily functions.
Importance in Health
Each macronutrient has specific functions:
Carbohydrates - Main energy source for the body and essential for brain function.
Proteins - Crucial for muscle repair and growth, hormone production, and immune function.
Fats - Necessary for hormone production, absorption of fat-soluble vitamins, and providing sustained energy.
Role in Weight Loss
Balancing macronutrient intake helps control hunger, manage energy levels, and maintain muscle mass during weight loss.

Micronutrients

Vitamins and Minerals
Micronutrients are required in smaller amounts but are essential for various physiological processes, including metabolism, immune function, and cellular repair.
Importance in Health
Micronutrients contribute to bone health, immune function, energy production, and protection against oxidative stress.
Role in Weight Loss
Ensuring adequate intake of micronutrients supports overall health, which is crucial for sustained weight loss and optimal metabolism.
To calculate personal macro targets for weight loss, you can follow these general steps:

Determine Total Daily Energy Expenditure (TDEE)
TDEE represents the total number of calories your body burns in a day, including basal metabolic rate (BMR) and activity level.
Several online calculators or formulas can help estimate TDEE based on factors like age, gender, weight, height, and activity level.
Set Caloric Deficit
To lose weight, you typically need to consume fewer calories than your TDEE, creating a caloric deficit.
A moderate deficit of 500 to 750 calories per day is often recommended for safe and sustainable weight loss.

Distribute Macronutrients
Once you have your calorie target, you can allocate macronutrients based on recommended ranges.
Proteins: 0.8-1.0 grams per pound of body weight
Protein intake is crucial for muscle repair, growth, and overall

metabolic health. Consuming 0.8-1.0 grams of protein per pound of body weight helps support muscle mass preservation and satiety during weight loss.

Carbohydrates: 25-35% of daily intake

Carbohydrates provide energy and are essential for optimal brain function and physical performance. By consuming 25-35% of total calories from carbohydrates, you can still meet your energy needs while moderating intake for weight loss goals.

Fats: Remaining percentage of total calories

Fats are vital for hormone regulation, cell structure, and nutrient absorption. The remaining percentage of daily calories not allocated to protein and carbohydrates can come from fats, typically ranging from 20-35% of total calorie intake.

4. **Adjust Based on Goals and Preferences**

Fine-tune your macronutrient distribution based on personal preferences, dietary restrictions, and fitness goals.

Experiment with different ratios to find what works best for your body and lifestyle.

Consulting with a registered dietitian or nutritionist can provide personalised guidance and ensure your macronutrient targets align with your health and weight loss objectives.

6

Sample Recipes

Breakfast

Smoked Salmon Omlette

Serves 1

- 4oz (112g) Cottage Cheese
- 40g Finely Chopped Spinach
- 2 Eggs & 1/2 Cup Egg Whites
- 1/4 Cup Milk (any type)
- 2 tsp. Mixed Herbs Or Your Favourite Spices
- 3.5 oz. (100g) Smoked Salmon, Chopped

Place the cottage cheese in a bowl and mix with the hand blender (or food processor) until smooth.

Beat the eggs, egg whites with the milk and herbs/spices in a separate bowl.

Spray or oil and heat the frying pan, fry the egg mixture over medium heat for 2 minutes until the egg solidifies, add spinach, fold omelette then turn over. Fry the other side for 1-2 minutes or until desired texture is reached.

To serve, spread the cottage cheese paste over the omelette and top with smoked salmon.

Protein Blueberry Pancakes

Serves 1

- 1/4 Cup Egg Whites (around 4 eggs)
- 1 Scoop (25g) Of Vanilla Whey Powder
- 1/2 Banana, Mashed
- Almond milk, If needed
- 1/4 Cup (25g) Fresh Or Frozen Blueberries
- 1/2 tsp. Coconut Oil

Whisk together the egg whites and protein powder. Stir in the mashed banana and add the blueberries. If the pancake mixture seems too thick, add a splash of almond milk to thin it.

Heat the coconut oil in a pan to low-medium. Pour in the pancake mixture and cook until little bubbles form (about 5 minutes). Make sure the pancake has set enough before you try flipping it, then flip over. Cook the pancake for another 2-3 minutes.

Lunch

Grilled Chicken & Pineapple Spinach Salad

Serves 1

For The Salad:

- 5oz (125g) Chicken Breast
- 3 Slices Pineapple, Canned
- 2 Handfuls Spinach
- 1/4 Cup Mint Leaves
- 1/4 Small Onion, Finely Chopped

For the Dressing:

- 1 Tbsp Olive Oil
- 1 Tsp Ginger, Grated
- 1 Clove Garlic, Minced
- 1/2 Lime, Juiced
- 1 Tsp Honey
- Tabasco, Optional

Mix the ingredients of the dressing in a salad bowl, season with salt. Add in the spinach and mint leaves and let it rest.

In the meantime, cut the chicken breast in half, place on a hot grill pan, and cover each chicken with slices of pineapple, season with black pepper. Grill for around 6-8 minutes, then turn and grill for another 5 minutes (at this stage remove the pineapple and let it grill next to the chicken). Make sure the chicken reaches 165 degree internal temp before removing from the pan. Remove from the heat and let the chicken rest for 3 minutes, then cut it into strips.

Add the chicken to the salad together with sliced pineapple and finely chopped onion, mix before serving.

**Vegetarian option: replace the grilled chicken with fried or baked tofu.

Protein Quinoa Bowl (Vegan)

Serves 2

For the Bowl:

- 1 Medium Sweet Potato, Sliced Or Diced
- 1 Tablespoon Oil
- 1/4 Cup Uncooked Quinoa
- 4 Cups Kale, Chopped
- 1 Cup Edamame
- 1 Ripe Avocado, Diced
- Sunflower Seeds, For Topping
- Hemp Hearts, For Fopping
- Nutritional Yeast, For topping
- Salt to taste

For the Dressing:

- 2 Tablespoons Tahini
- 1 Teaspoon Low Sodium Soy Sauce
- 1 Teaspoon White Wine Vinegar
- 1 Small Garlic Clove, Finely Grated

- 1-2 Tablespoons Water As Needed

Preheat the oven to 400ºF.

Prepare the sweet potato, place on a baking sheet and drizzle with oil. Toss to cover evenly and sprinkle with salt to taste. Roast for 30 minutes at 400ºF or until tender and lightly golden.

Meanwhile, add the quinoa in a small saucepan with 1/2 cup of water. Bring to a boil, then reduce heat and simmer covered for 15 minutes or until the water has been absorbed.

Once the quinoa is cooked, add the frozen edamame to the quinoa and cover. The steam should thaw and warm the edamame. Set aside. Chop the kale and divide into 2 bowls.

Prepare the dressing, in a small bowl or jar, whisk together all the ingredients except for the water. The mixture should be thick. Add water as needed, 1/2 tablespoon at a time. The dressing should be creamy and easy to drizzle.

Assemble the salad, top the kale with the quinoa and edamame. Add the roasted sweet potato. Drizzle with the dressing and top with avocado, sunflower seeds, hemp hearts and nutritional yeast.

Dinner

Miso Salmon With Zucchini Noodles

Serves 2

For the salmon:

- 2 Salmon Fillets, 4.5 oz. (130g) Each
- 2 Tbsp Miso Paste
- 2 Tbsp Honey

- 1/4 Cup Tamari, Or Soy Sauce
- 2 Tbsp Ginger, Grated
- 2 Tbsp Apple Cider Vinegar
- 1 Tbsp Sesame Oil
- 2 Tsp Sesame Seeds

For the noodles:

- 14 Oz (400g) Zucchini Noodles
- 6 Radishes, Sliced
- 2 Tsp Sesame Oil
- 2 Tsp Ginger, Grated
- 1 Tsp Honey
- 2 Tbsp Soy Sauce
- Juice Of 1 Lime

Mix all the salmon marinade ingredients. Coat the salmon fillets in the marinade and refrigerate for at least 20 minutes.

In the meantime, place the zucchini noodles and sliced radish in a bowl. Mix all the ingredients for the dressing and pour over the salad. Mix well and refrigerate.

Preheat the oven to 350°F (180°C).

Place the salmon in an oven safe dish and pour some of the marinade over it. Bake for 12 minutes and then turn the broiler on for about 2-3 minutes to brown the top.

Check often to avoid burning. Once cooked, serve salmon alongside the zucchini salad. Sprinkle with sesame seeds to serve.

Turkey & Broccoli Stir-Fry

Serves 2

- 3.5 oz. (100g) Rice Noodles
- 7 oz. (200g) Turkey Fillet, Chopped
- 1 Head Broccoli, Diced Into Florets
- 1 Tbsp Olive Oil
- 4 Tbsp Soy Sauce Or Tamari
- 2 Tsp Sesame Oil
- 1 Tbsp Rice Vinegar
- 1 Tbsp Grated Ginger
- 2 Tbsp Spring Onion, Chopped
- Handful Coriander, To Serve

Cook the noodles according to the instructions on the packaging. Strain and rinse with cold water, then set aside. In a wok or deep pan, heat the olive oil and fry the turkey for about 3-4 minutes. Add in the broccoli florets and fry for another 1-2 minutes. Next, pour half a cup of water and 3 tbsp. of soy sauce, then cook until all the water evaporates and the broccoli is tender (about 10 minutes).

In the meantime, mix together the remaining soy sauce, sesame oil, vinegar, grated ginger, and mix well. Once turkey and broccoli are ready, add in the cooked noodles and heat it for 2-3 minutes. Take off the heat, pour in the sauce and gently mix.

Serve with chopped spring onions and coriander leaves.

7

Exercise Tailored to Your Lifestyle

In the pursuit of a healthy lifestyle, exercise stands as a cornerstone, offering a multitude of benefits beyond just physical appearance. It is the foundational pillar upon which we build resilience, vitality, and longevity. However, understanding that exercise isn't a one-size-fits-all endeavour is crucial. It's about aligning your regimen with your fitness level, age, and personal goals.

Understanding Your Fitness Level, Age, and Goals

Before delving into the specifics of exercise, it's essential to acknowledge that each individual's journey is unique. Factors like age, current fitness level, and personal objectives play pivotal roles in crafting an effective workout routine.

Fitness Level: Whether you're a seasoned athlete or just embarking on your fitness journey, it's imperative to start at a level that challenges you without overwhelming your body. Gradual progression is key to preventing injuries and ensuring sustainable results.

Age: Aging brings about changes in our bodies, necessitating modifications in our exercise routines. While younger individuals may focus on high-intensity workouts, older adults may benefit more from low-impact activities that preserve joint health while improving strength and flexibility.

Goals: Your fitness goals serve as guiding beacons, shaping the direction of your exercise regimen. Whether it's weight loss, muscle gain, enhanced endurance, or overall well-being, tailoring your workouts to these objectives optimises your chances of success.

The Importance of 8000 Steps Per Day and Hydration

Walking, often overlooked as a form of exercise, holds tremendous benefits for individuals of all ages and fitness levels. Striving to achieve 8000 steps per day serves as a simple yet effective way to incorporate physical activity into your daily routine. It enhances cardiovascular health, boosts metabolism, and fosters mental well-being.

In tandem with regular movement, adequate hydration is paramount. Water is the elixir of life, facilitating nutrient transportation, temperature regulation, and waste removal within the body. Aim to consume at least eight glasses of water daily, adjusting based on individual needs and activity levels.

The Equilibrium of Strength Training and Cardio for Fat Loss

Dispelling the myth that cardio reigns supreme in the realm of fat loss, strength training emerges as an indispensable ally. While cardiovascular exercises burn calories during the workout, strength training cultivates lean muscle mass, elevating your resting metabolic rate and promoting fat loss even at rest.

Striking a harmonious balance between strength training and cardio optimises fat loss while sculpting a lean, toned physique. Incorporating both modalities into your exercise routine ensures comprehensive development, fostering resilience and functional fitness.

Sample Home-Based Workouts

Low-Intensity Workout
1. Warm-Up (5 minutes)
Begin with dynamic stretches targeting major muscle groups.
2. Bodyweight Circuit (15 minutes)
Perform 10-12 reps of squats, push-ups, lunges, and planks with 30 seconds rest between each exercise.
3. Cardio Finisher (10 minutes)
Engage in brisk walking, jogging in place, or dancing to elevate heart rate.
4. Cool Down and Stretch (5 minutes)
Conclude with static stretches to enhance flexibility and reduce muscle tension.

Medium-Intensity Workout

1. Warm-Up (7 minutes) Incorporate dynamic movements such as arm circles, leg swings, and torso twists.
2. Resistance Band Circuit (20 minutes)

Utilise resistance bands for exercises like bicep curls, lateral raises, squats, and rows, performing 12-15 reps per set.
3. Interval Training (15 minutes)
Alternate between one-minute bursts of high-intensity exercises (jumping jacks, mountain climbers) and one-minute active recovery (walking or jogging in place).
4. Cooldown and Mobility Work (8 minutes)
Conclude with foam rolling and gentle stretches to enhance recovery and mobility.

Sample Gym-Based Workouts

Low-Intensity Workout
1. Warm-Up (7 minutes)
Utilise cardio machines like the treadmill or elliptical for a gradual warm-up.
2. Machine Circuit (20 minutes)
Engage in resistance exercises using machines targeting major muscle groups with moderate weights and 12-15 reps per set.
3. Walking or Cycling (15 minutes)
Maintain a steady pace on the treadmill or stationary bike to sustain heart rate elevation.
4. Stretching and Flexibility (8 minutes)
Dedicate time to static stretching, focusing on areas of tightness and discomfort.

Medium-Intensity Workout
1. Warm-Up (10 minutes)
Incorporate dynamic movements and foam rolling to prepare the body for exertion.
2. Free Weight Circuit (25 minutes)
Perform compound exercises like squats, deadlifts, bench presses, and rows with challenging weights and 8-10 reps per set.
3. HIIT Cardio (15 minutes)
Alternate between sprints on the treadmill or rowing machine and active recovery periods.
4. Core Strengthening (10 minutes)
Integrate exercises like planks, Russian twists, and leg raises to target the core musculature.
5. Cooldown and Stretch (10 minutes)
Conclude with deep breathing and comprehensive stretching to

facilitate recovery and prevent soreness.

Conclusion

On the path to a healthy lifestyle, exercise emerges as a vibrant thread, weaving together vitality, resilience, and longevity. By embracing a holistic approach tailored to your fitness level, age, and goals, you unlock the transformative power of movement. From the simplicity of daily steps to the intricacies of strength training and cardio, each facet contributes to the mosaic of your well-being. Embrace the journey, honouring your body's unique needs and aspirations, as you embark on the path to holistic health and vitality.

8

A Roadmap To Lasting Health and Happiness

Congratulations on reaching the conclusion of this transformative journey. Your commitment to delving into these pages is a testament to your dedication to living a healthier, happier, and more balanced life.

As you reflect on the insights and strategies shared throughout this book, remember that knowledge is only as powerful as the actions we take based on it. Each idea, each suggestion, is a stepping stone toward creating the life you envision—one filled with vitality, fulfilment, and purpose.

Implementing these strategies into your daily routine may require effort and patience, but know that every small change you make is a step forward on your path to wellness. Whether it's adopting mindfulness practices, nourishing your body with wholesome foods, prioritising self-care, or fostering meaningful connections, each decision contributes to your overall well-being.

It's important to acknowledge that progress is not always linear. There will be days of triumph and days of challenge, but it's in these moments of struggle that growth truly occurs. Be gentle with yourself, celebrate your successes, and learn from your setbacks.

Remember, the journey to a healthier, happier, and more balanced life is ongoing. Embrace the process, stay committed to your goals, and trust in your ability to create positive change.

As you close this chapter and embark on the next phase of your journey, know that you are well-equipped with the tools and insights to thrive. May you continue to cultivate joy, cultivate gratitude, and cultivate love in every aspect of your life.

Here's to the beautiful adventure that lies ahead—a life filled with abundance, vitality, and purpose. Congratulations on taking this important step toward your best self.

Your journey awaits—embrace it with open arms and an open heart.